Divine Healing

Prayer

Pray this Prayer for Your Healing

Joel & Heidi Hitchcock

TABLE OF CONTENTS

Dedication

To our Lord Jesus Christ – the LORD our Healer.

A few years back, a local group hosted a *health and wholeness fair* in a nearby town, and offered vendors a table for a fee.

Heidi and I thought about it, and decided to rent one of those tables to present our belief that physical and emotional healing comes from the LORD.

We already knew that there would be many *new age* presentations too, which we strongly dismiss because of our belief in Jesus and the Bible. However, we saw in this event a good opportunity to share the LORD.

We did not have much time, so I dedicated about a day or two drafting a little document, "Divine Healing Prayer." In it I wrote a prayer based on Bible verses that were relevant to healing.

We then printed it out on our little printer in our home. To give it some respectability, we bound each one in clear plastic covers with white, slide-off spines.

When we got to the fair, we discovered exactly what we expected. There were *healers* of every shade. Little Buddhas and other meditating sculptures overlooked the buzz of activity presented by yogists, herbalists, massagists, and many other nice people.

This was not our typical revival service! But Heidi took the lead, and I supported her. She set up her table, set a chair beside it, with an invitation for prayer. Several people showed some interest, sat on the chair, and let Heidi pray a simple prayer of faith and love over them, anointing them with oil.

Each one also received a copy of the *Divine Healing Prayer.*

What I witnessed was amazing. The Holy Spirit came! I could see the effects of His Presence on some of them, as tears began to stream down their cheeks. One lady was so touched that she wanted to come see us again. She told us about how her physical pain left her during our prayer.

It was a wonderful opportunity to share the love of Jesus with those dear people.

We had several copies of the *Divine Healing Prayer* left, which we gave to friends or to whoever else might be benefitted by it. I did not expect such a positive response. So many people requested a copy for them, or for their friends.

Though I don't think I always get it right, there is a little perfectionist inside of me, which is a blessing (because I always want to reflect a spirit of excellence for the Lord,) but sometimes it is a hindrance, because it may keep me from putting something into print when I do not have all the *t's* crossed and *i's* dotted.

This little booklet is an example of it. I have always wanted to write an extensive healing prayer book (like I did for financial provision,[1]) but time and other pressing things have kept me from it. Maybe I will do such an extensive one sometime in the future.

But a couple of weeks ago, I yet again received a request for a copy of the *Divine Healing Prayer*. That got me started.

------

[1] "Effectual Fervent Prayers for God's Abundant Provision," by Joel Hitchcock, available on Amazon or www.joelhitchcock.blogspot.com.

With the old draft by my side, I typed out every single word again, changed a little here and there, added the related Scripture verses in the footnotes, and made it available in this little booklet you are holding in your hands right now.

Although it is a *simple* prayer, and lacks a little *sophistication,* they say, if it works, leave it as is.

I pray that you will be mightily blessed, and healed as you use it in your prayer times.

May I also give a little instruction regarding medicine and your medical professionals. This booklet does not suggest that medication and professional medical help should be discarded.

And finally, please remember to always trust God in both sickness and in health. The *healing evangelist* in my urges you to receive your healing, in Jesus' Name. The *pastor* in me comforts you to not give up hope and faith if your healing does not manifest, whether right away or in time. Do not allow disappointments to discourage you. God is God and He is our Sovereign Lord, and He is our Loving Father. Keep your trust in God. He knows what He is doing. God is working, even in our hardest times. The LORD is your Shepherd, and He is with you through it all.

Introduction

The Bible teaches us that healing is available for our entire being – body, soul, and spirit.[2]

Healing in the Atonement

This healing is provided for us in the atonement, (what Jesus wrought in His powerful death and resurrection.) Peter wrote, Who in His own self bare our sins in his own body on the tree [the cross,] that we being dead to sins, should live unto righteousness: by whose stripes ye were healed" (1 Peter, 2:24, KJV.)

---

[2] "Now may the God of peace Himself sanctify you completely; and may your whole spirit, soul, and body be preserved blameless at the coming of our Lord Jesus Christ" (1 Thessalonians 5:23.) In this booklet, I have used the words *soul* and *spirit* interchangeably, to refer to our inner self.

Healing in and from God's Word

It also says, He sent His Word and healed their diseases" (Psalm 107:20, KJV.)

God is a God of His Word. When He says something, it is considered a promise. He is a Promise-Keeping God.

"For all the promises of God in him *are* yea, and in him Amen, unto the glory of God by us" (1 Corinthians 1:20, KJV.)

"God *is* not a man, that he should lie; neither the son of man, that he should repent: hath he said, and shall he not do *it*? or hath he spoken, and shall he not make it good?" (Number 23:19, KJV.)

God's Word will not return to Him void. "So shall my Word be that goeth forth out of my mouth: it shall not return unto me void, but it shall accomplish that which I please, and it shall prosper in the thing whereto I sent it" (Isaiah 55:11, KJV.)

God is eager to honor His Word. "Thou hast well seen: for I will hasten My Word to perform it" (Jeremiah 1:12, KJV.)

There is power in thoughts and words

The Bible also teaches that there is power in our thoughts and words. When we think and speak life and healing over our bodies, we can expect miracles!

About our thoughts it says, "As a man thinketh in his heart, so is he" (Proverbs 23:7, KJV.)

About our words it says, "Death and life are in the power of the tongue. Them that love it shall eat the fruit thereof" (Proverbs 18:21, KJV.)

Our words can move the mountains of sickness and disease. Jesus said, "For verily I say unto you, That whosoever shall say unto this mountain, Be thou removed, and be thou cast into the sea; and shall not doubt in his heart, but shall believe that those things which he saith shall come to pass; he shall have whatsoever he saith" (Mark 11:23, KJV.)

The Divine Healing Prayer

This *Divine Healing Prayer* is intended to instill and release *thoughts of healing* into your heart, and help you use the power of the tongue by saying, declaring, and confessing the promises of the *Omnipotent Healer*, as found in the Bible.

The thoughts and words in themselves do not heal. It is *the One* who gave the promises, who heals, and He is with you this very moment. His wonderful Presence is manifested when you focus on Him and reveal faith in Him. It is not your faith that heals, but faith draws on the power of *the One* who heals.

How to Use the Divine Healing Prayer

You may read this *Divine Healing Prayer* as many times as you wish, until it flows freely from your heart, and lips. Once a week, once a day, twice a day, first thing in the morning, or before you retire at night, or in whichever way your schedule allows.

While praying, you should focus on the *words and thoughts,* and more importantly, focus on *the One* to whom your prayer is prayed. As you pray, the Spirit will come. His Presence may manifest as a warm sensation, like heat upon your body. This Presence should not be feared. Welcome Him! The more He is welcomed, the stronger His power will manifest. This sensation is known as *the anointing,* the term for *the tangible presence and power of God.*

THE DIVINE HEALING PRAYER (LONGER)

"My Dear Loving Heavenly Father,

I approach You this day, in the Name of Your Son, Jesus Christ. I thank You today for the wonderful privilege I have, that I may come into Your Presence without guilt of fear (Hebrews 10:19-22, KJV.)[3]

Today, I refuse to focus on my disease. I do not deny the existence of my disease, but I do deny its right to exist in my body. I will not be focused on the disease. Rather, I will focus on the LORD, and on Your healing power in me. Greater is He

---

[3] "Having therefore, brethren, boldness to enter into the holiest by the blood of Jesus, By a new and living way, which he hath consecrated for us, through the veil, that is to say, his flesh; And having an high priest over the house of God; Let us draw near with a true heart in full assurance of faith, having our hearts sprinkled from an evil conscience, and our bodies washed with pure water" (Hebrews 10:19-22, KJV.)

that is in me, than he that is in the world (1 John 4:4, KJV.) [4]

Jesus, You died on the cross for my sins and sickness. You were wounded for my transgressions. You were bruised for my iniquities. The chastisement of my peace was upon You and with Your stripes I am healed (Isaiah 53:5, KJV.)[5]

Lord, You sent Your Word, and healed my diseases (Psalm 107:20, KJV.) [6] Your Word shall

---

[4] "Ye are of God, little children, and have overcome them: because greater is he that is in you, than he that is in the world" (1 John 4:4, KJV.)

[5] "But he was wounded for our transgressions, he was bruised for our iniquities: the chastisement of our peace was upon him; and with his stripes we are healed" (Isaiah 54:5, KJV.)

[6] "He sent his word, and healed them, and delivered them from their destructions" (Psalm 107:20, KJV.)

not return to You void, but it shall accomplish its sent purpose (Isaiah 55:11.)[7]

You are *Yahweh Rapha*, the LORD that healeth me (Exodus 15:26.)[8]

Today I refuse to focus on my disease. I do not deny the existence of the disease, but I do indeed deny its right to exist in my body. I consider not my own body, I stagger not at the promise of God through unbelief; but I am strong in faith, giving glory to God; And being fully persuaded

---

[7] For as the rain cometh down, and the snow from heaven, and returneth not thither, but watereth the earth, and maketh it bring forth and bud, that it may give seed to the sower, and bread to the eater: So shall my word be that goeth forth out of my mouth: it shall not return unto me void, but it shall accomplish that which I please, and it shall prosper in the thing whereto I sent it" (Isaiah 55:10-11, KJV.)

[8] "And said, If thou wilt diligently hearken to the voice of the Lord thy God, and wilt do that which is right in his sight, and wilt give ear to his commandments, and keep all his statutes, I will put none of these diseases upon thee, which I have brought upon the Egyptians: for I am the Lord that healeth thee" (Exodus 15:26, KJV.)

that, what You have promised, You are able also to perform (Romans 4:19-21.) [9]

I focus not on the disease, but rather on the LORD, and in Your healing power within me, for greater is He that is in me, than he that is in the world (1 John 4:4.)

As Abraham believed in Him who raises the dead, and calls those things that be not as though they were, I too call forth my healing, even before it manifests in the natural (Romans 4:17.) Against [no] hope, I too believe in hope, according to that

---

[9] "And being not weak in faith, he considered not his own body now dead, when he was about an hundred years old, neither yet the deadness of Sara's womb: He staggered not at the promise of God through unbelief; but was strong in faith, giving glory to God; And being fully persuaded that, what he had promised, he was able also to perform" (Romans 4:19-21, KJV.)

which was spoken [or written in Your Word] (Romans 4:18.)[10]

As I think in my heart, so am I (Proverbs 23:7.)[11] Therefore, I think of myself well, according to Your promises. You said death and life are in the power of my tongue (Proverbs 18:21.)

Therefore, I will not allow my tongue to habitually speak words of death and disease. Rather, I will speak life, for death *and* life are in the power of the tongue. I will speak words of health and healing, as I am doing this moment.

These words of health and healing have a healing effect upon my body and soul. If I say

---

[10] Romans 4:17-18, KJV.)

[11] "For as he thinketh in his heart, so *is* he…" (Proverbs 23:7, KJV.)

something, and do so with faith, miracles are waiting to happen on my behalf.

I have faith *in* God and I possess the faith *of* God[12] – the *God-kind of faith.* I say unto this mountain to be removed and be cast into the sea.

I do not doubt in my heart, but believe that whatsoever I say will come to pass, and that I will have whatsoever I say. Whatever it is that I desire, when I pray, I believe that I receive it, and in due time, I will receive it in the natural realm (Mark 11:22-24.)[13]

---

[12] "Yeshua answered and he said to them, "May the faith of God be in you" (Mark 11:22, ABPB.)

[13] And Jesus answering saith unto them, Have faith in God. For verily I say unto you, That whosoever shall say unto this mountain, Be thou removed, and be thou cast into the sea; and shall not doubt in his heart, but shall believe that those things which he saith shall come to pass; he shall have whatsoever he saith. Therefore I say unto you, What things soever ye desire, when ye pray, believe that ye receive *them*, and ye shall have *them.*

My healing first becomes a reality in my spirit, then a reality in my body.

It is Your will for me to be healed, for You said, "I will, be thou clean" (Matthew 8:3.)[14]

It is Your will to heal me, because Your will is revealed in Your Word. I am your beloved, and You wish above all things that I prosper and be in health, even as my soul prospers (3 John 2.)[15]

Sickness is not the will of my Loving Creator. It was the adversary that went forth and smote Job with boils from the soles of his foot unto his crown (Joh 2:7.)[16]

---

[14] "And Jesus put forth *his* hand, and touched him, saying, I will; be thou clean. And immediately his leprosy was cleansed" (Matthew 8:3, KJV.)

[15] "Beloved, I wish above all things that thou mayest prosper and be in health, even as thy soul prospereth" (3 John 2, KJV.)

[16] "So went Satan forth from the presence of the LORD, and smote Job with sore boils from the sole of his foot unto his crown. And he took him a

But You turned the captivity of Job,[17] and You deliver me also, for You are the LORD that healeth me (Exodus 15:26.)

I will not allow fear,[18] for You have not given me a spirit of fear, but of power, and of love, and of a sound mind (2 Timothy 1:7.)[19] My mind is sound, because it is focused on You and Your promises.

I will not be doubleminded, for a doubleminded man is unstable in all of his ways.

------

potsherd to scrape himself withal; and he sat down among the ashes." (Job 2:7-8, KJV.)

[17] "And the LORD turned the captivity of Job, when he prayed for his friends: also the LORD gave Job twice as much as he had before" (Job 42:10, KJV.)

[18] "For the thing which I greatly feared is come upon me, and that which I was afraid of is come unto me" (Job 3:25, KJV.)

[19] "For God hath not given us the spirit of fear; but of power, and of love, and of a sound mind" (2 Timothy 1:7, KJV.)

Let not such a man think that he shall receive anything from the Lord (James 1:5-8.)[20] Therefore, I shall be *single-minded,* focused on Your Word. I shall not allow fear to steal my faith and hope.

For faith is the substance of things hoped for – the evidence of things not seen. I too receive a good report by my faith in God.[21] Regardless of my medical report, I believe the report of the Lord – the report of Your Word.

I can see what can be, for I can see the unseen. By faith I understand the worlds were framed by the Word of God, and material, seen things were

---

[20] "If any of you lack wisdom, let him ask of God, that giveth to all *men* liberally, and upbraideth not; and it shall be given him. But let him ask in faith, nothing wavering. For he that wavereth is like a wave of the sea driven with the wind and tossed. For let not that man think that he shall receive any thing of the Lord. A double minded man *is* unstable in all his ways" (James 1:5-8, KJV.)

[21] "Now faith is the substance of things hoped for, the evidence of things not seen. For by it the elders obtained a good report" (Hebrews 11:1-2, KJV.)

not made of material, visible things (Hebrews 11:3.)[22] By faith, I can see myself healed and whole.

Without faith it is impossible to please God, but he that cometh to God must believe that He is, and that He is a rewarder of them that diligently seek You (Hebrews 11:6.)[23]

Though my situation may seem impossible, I am not ruled by the laws of disease and oppression (Romans 8:2.)[24] I am ruled by another law, another principle, for I have been translated from the

----

[22] "Through faith we understand that the worlds were framed by the word of God, so that things which are seen were not made of things which do appear" (Hebrews 11:3, KJV.)

[23] "But without faith *it is* impossible to please *him*: for he that cometh to God must believe that he is, and *that* he is a rewarder of them that diligently seek him" (Hebrews 11:6, KJV.)

[24] "For the law of the Spirit of life in Christ Jesus hath made me free from the law of sin and death" (Romans 8:2, KJV.)

kingdom of darkness into the Kingdom of Your dear Son (Colossians 1:13, KJV.)[25] I am no longer a subject of the kingdom of darkness, disease, and fear. I am a citizen of the Kingdom of Heaven, and I have access to all the rights of a duly accepted citizen Your Kingdom. I once was far off, but have been made nigh by the Blood of Jesus (Ephesians 2:13.)[26]

Oh God, nothing is impossible with you. With man it may be impossible, but not with God, for with God all things are possible (Mark 10:17.)[27]

---

[25] Who hath delivered us from the power of darkness, and hath translated *us* into the kingdom of his dear Son:

[26] "But now in Christ Jesus ye who sometimes were far off are made nigh by the blood of Christ" (Ephesians 2:13, KJV.)

[27] "And Jesus looking upon them saith, With men *it is* impossible, but not with God: for with God all things are possible" (Mark 10:27, KJV.)

The LORD is my helper, and I will not fear what man shall do unto me (Hebrews 13:6.)[28]

Behold, You are the LORD, the God of all flesh: Is there anything too hard for You? Oh, LORD, behold, thou hast made the heaven and the earth by thy great power and stretched out arm, and there is nothing too hard for thee… (Jeremiah 32:17, 27.)[29]

I believe You and Your promises, and I expect miracles to happen, for with God nothing shall be impossible (Luke 1:37.)[30]

---

[28] "So that we may boldly say, The Lord *is* my helper, and I will not fear what man shall do unto me" (Hebrews 13:6, KJV.)

[29] Behold, I *am* the LORD, the God of all flesh: is there any thing too hard for me?" (Jeremiah 32:27, KJV,) "Ah Lord GOD! behold, thou hast made the heaven and the earth by thy great power and stretched out arm, *and* there is nothing too hard for thee" (Jeremiah 32:17, KJV.)

[30] For with God nothing shall be impossible.

The One who can cause a virgin to conceive, can also cause me to conceive a unique miracle, manifested in my own body and soul.

If You could heal an entire nation in a single day, You can certainly heal me also! You brought them forth with silver and gold: and there was not one feeble person among their tribes (Psalm 105:37.)[31]

Lord Jesus, You healed entire multitudes (Luke 6:19,)[32] and You can certainly heal me too.

They sought to touch You, for healing virtue flowed from You, and Your healing power flows into me also. I reach out and touch You with my

-----

[31] "He brought them forth also with silver and gold: and *there was* not one feeble *person* among their tribes" (Psalm 105:37, KJV.)

[32] "And the whole multitude sought to touch him: for there went virtue out of him, and healed them all" (Luke 6:19, KJV.)

hope and faith. Healing virtue and miracle working power comes forth from You and makes me whole by my faith in You (Mark 5:30, 34.)[33]

I open myself up to the free flow of Your mighty power into my life.

God, You anointed Jesus of Nazareth with the Holy Spirit and with power, and He went about doing good and healing all that were oppressed of the devil, for God was with Him (Acts 10:38.)[34]

Your sweet anointing is Your tangible presence and power. I allow that Presence, that glorious power to flow through my body. This very

---

[33] "And Jesus, immediately knowing in himself that virtue had gone out of him, turned him about in the press, and said, Who touched my clothes?" (Matthew 5:30, KJV.) "And he said unto her, Daughter, thy faith hath made thee whole; go in peace, and be whole of thy plague (Mark 5:34, KJV.)

[34] "How God anointed Jesus of Nazareth with the Holy Ghost and with power: who went about doing good, and healing all that were oppressed of the devil; for God was with him" (Acts 10:38, KJV.)

moment I become aware of Your power surging through my body and soul. A warm sensation of Your beautiful presence envelops me. It is like a blanket of love that is wrapped about me. A sensation like electricity softly and gently goes through my body. The sensation become stronger and stronger, and I am overwhelmed with a sense of Your mighty love and power.

If the power of God was present even in the bones of a prophet, and caused a dead man to come back to life, how much the more may the power of God raise me to health while I am still living (2 Kings 13:21.)[35]

---

[35] "And it came to pass, as they were burying a man, that, behold, they spied a band of men; and they cast the man into the sepulchre of Elisha: and when the man was let down, and touched the bones of Elisha, he revived, and stood up on his feet" (2 Kings 13:21, KJV.)

I shall not die, but live, and declare the works of the Lord! (Psalm 118:17.)[36]

Lord, I have prayed the effectual, fervent prayer of the righteous – a prayer energized by the Holy Spirit. This kind of prayer availeth much, and has great results. I pray, and I accept the prayers of mature believers, anointing me, and praying over me in the Name of the Lord. And the prayer of faith shall save the sick, and if he hath committed any sin, it shall be forgiven him (James 5:14-16.)[37]

---

[36] "I shall not die, but live, and declare the works of the LORD" (Psalm 118:17, KJV.)

[37] "Is any sick among you? let him call for the elders of the church; and let them pray over him, anointing him with oil in the name of the Lord: And the prayer of faith shall save the sick, and the Lord shall raise him up; and if he have committed sins, they shall be forgiven him. Confess *your* faults one to another, and pray one for another, that ye may be healed. The effectual fervent prayer of a righteous man availeth much" (James 5:14-16, KJV.)

I repent of my sin. For sin is a hindrance to the free flow of the power of God. If I keep sin in my heart, the Lord will not hear me (Psalm 66:18.)[38] But if I confess my sin, You are faithful and just to forgive me of my sin, and cleanse me from all unrighteousness (1 John 1:9.)[39]

I forgive men their trespasses, and my Heavenly Father forgives me too (Matthew 6:14.)[40]

I will not serve two masters.[41] I serve the One God (Deuteronomy 6:4-5,)[42] for this is eternal life

---

[38] "If I regard iniquity in my heart, the Lord will not hear me" (Psalm 66:18, KJV.)

[39] "If we confess our sins, he is faithful and just to forgive us *our* sins, and to cleanse us from all unrighteousness" (1 John 1:9, KJV.)

[40] "For if you forgive men their trespasses, your heavenly Father will also forgive you" (Matthew 6:14, KJV.)

[41] Matthew 6:24, 1 Kings 18:21, 1 Samuel 5:1-7, Joshua 24:15.

[42] "Hear, O Israel: The LORD our God *is* one LORD. And thou shalt love the LORD thy God with all thine heart, and with all thy soul, and with all thy might" (Deuteronomy 6:5-6, KJV.)

– to believe in You, the Only True God, and Jesus Christ whom thou hast sent (John 17:3.)[43] I shalt worship no other god: for the LORD, whose name *is* Jealous, *is* a jealous God (Exodus 34:14.)[44]

Therefore, I accept Jesus today, either for the first time, or I do so again, confirming that You are my Lord and my Savior.

Jesus, You stand at the door and know. I hear Your voice and open the door, and You come in and dine with me, and me with thee (Revelation

---

[43] "And this is life eternal, that they might know thee the only true God, and Jesus Christ, whom thou hast sent (John 17:3, KJV.)

[44] "For thou shalt worship no other god: for the LORD, whose name *is* Jealous, *is* a jealous God" (Exodus 34:14, KJV.)

3:20.)[45] I ask for forgiveness, wash me of my sins in Your precious Blood (1 John 1:7.)[46]

I rely not on my own righteousness, for by Your holy standards, and in the brilliant light of Your glory, even my righteous deeds are as filthy rags. (Isaiah 64:6.)[47]

Rather, I rely on Jesus, and on His death and resurrection, to wash and cleanse me. Therefore, if any man be in Christ, he is a new creature: old things are passed away; behold, all things are

---

[45] "Behold, I stand at the door and knock; if anyone hears My voice and opens the door, I will come in to him and will dine with him, and he with Me" (Revelation 3:20, NASB.)

[46] "But if we walk in the light, as he is in the light, we have fellowship one with another, and the blood of Jesus Christ his Son cleanseth us from all sin" (1 John 1:7, KJV.)

[47] "But we are all as an unclean thing, and all our righteousnesses are as filthy rags; and we all do fade as a leaf; and our iniquities, like the wind, have taken us away" (Isaiah 64:6, KJV.)

become new (2 Corinthians 5:17.)[48] This moment, all things become new for me. You wash me with the water of Your Word and Spirit (Ephesians 5:26, KJV.)[49]

You anoint my head with oil, my cup runneth over. On the inside, I am clothed with a white robe of righteousness. Surely goodness and mercy shall follow me all the days of my life, and I will dwell in the house of the Lord forever (Psalm 23, Revelation 3:18.)

I receive my healing, and consider it done, in the mighty Name of Jesus. Because whatsoever I

---

[48] 2 Corinthians 5:17, KJV.

[49] "That he might sanctify and cleanse it with the washing of water by the word" (Ephesians 5:26, KJV.)

ask in Your Name, that You will do, that the Father may be glorified in the Son (John 14:13.)[50]

I will not give up hope and faith. I will keep on praying and believing, thanking, and praising, until and way beyond the day my miracle manifests in my body.

In Jesus' Name,

Amen.

---

[50] "And whatsoever ye shall ask in my name, that will I do, that the Father may be glorified in the Son" (John 14:13, KJV.)

The Divine Healing Prayer (Shorter)

Dear Father God,

Your Word says, "Beloved, I wish above all things that you may prosper in all things, and be in health, just as your soul prospers" (3 John 2, NKJV.)

I believe You are a better Father than any earthly parent could ever be. If no parent would wish sickness, disease, and oppression upon their child, how then would my Heavenly Father wish these things upon me.

Your word says, "Or what man is there among you who, if his son asks for bread, will give him a stone? Or if he asks for a fish, will he give him a serpent? If you then, being evil, know how to give good gifts to your children, how much more will your Father who is in heaven give good things to those who ask Him!" (Matthew 7:9-11.)

I therefore come to You with boldness and ask for healing in my body and in my soul.

Your Word teaches that, Whatsoever things I desire, when I pray, believe that I receive them, and I shall have them (Mark 11:23.)

I receive *the anointing* – the tangible power of God, that flows from Jesus. Oh, how God anointed Jesus of Nazareth with the Holy Spirit and with power, who went about doing good and healing all who were oppressed by the devil, for God was with Him (Acts 10:38, NKJV.)

Oh Lord, the whole multitude sought to touch You, for power went out from You and healed *them* all" ((Luke 6:19, NKJV.)

Your power was present to heal them, and Your power is present with me, this very moment, to heal me (Luke 5:17.) I reach out to touch You and You reach out to touch me. I receive that healing virtue right now.

Like a current of electricity, it flows through my body and soul. As it does, it brings life to my body. It kills disease in any form. It even energizes my immune system, and with prayer, exercise, and a healthy diet, I expect to live healthy. Your power flows into me and from me, and heals me from disease.

I accept Jesus as my Healer, my Lord, and My Savior. Wash my sins away with Your precious Blood, and make me white as snow. Give me a hunger for the things of God, and make Yourself more real to me than ever before (Revelation 3:20, Isaiah 1:18,[51] 1 John 1:7.)

I thank You for my healing.

In Jesus' Name,

Amen.

---

[51] "Come now, and let us reason together," Says the LORD, "Though your sins are like scarlet, They shall be as white as snow; Though they are red like crimson, They shall be as wool" (Isaiah 1:18, NKJV.)

You may pray this following prayer as a guideline: "Dear God. I am a sinner. I cannot save myself. I need a Savior, and Your Name is Jesus. Thank You God that You came to earth to reach me and to save me. Forgive me of all my sin and wash me clean with the precious blood of Jesus. I believe with my heart and confess with my mouth that Jesus died and rose again. I further declare that Jesus is my Lord from this day forward forever. You are my only God.

I open my life to you. Lord Jesus, come live in my heart. Please give me the power of Your Spirit that I may live righteously. Thank You for giving me eternal life, and that when I die, I will meet Jesus and live in heaven with You forever. Amen."

WHAT TO DO NOW?

Congratulations on receiving Jesus as your Lord and Savior! He now lives in your heart and you have received eternal life.

Now it is important that you grow in your faith and in your journey with God:

Tell several people that you have received Jesus Christ – not only will this one simple act give you a spiritual growth spurt, but it will give them an opportunity to receive Jesus too;

Be baptized by immersion, according to Matthew 28:19 and Acts 2:38 – in the Name of the Father, Son and Holy Spirit and in the Name of Jesus Christ;

Find a powerful, enthusiastic church that preaches the Bible without compromise, and attend it regularly;

Seek earnestly to be baptized in the Holy Spirit and power – which is a glorious experience accompanied by the speaking in tongues as in Acts 1:5-8 and 2:1-4;

Obtain a Bible (digital or paper,) and read it daily – if you read 3 chapters a day you will complete it in a year;

Pray daily – set aside a special time of your day for you and God, and also pray throughout the day (talk to God as if He is your friend;)

Refrain from old sinful habits like bad language and substance abuse – avoid the places and people who discourage your faith;

Make Christian friends that build you up and encourage you – they need you as much as you need them!

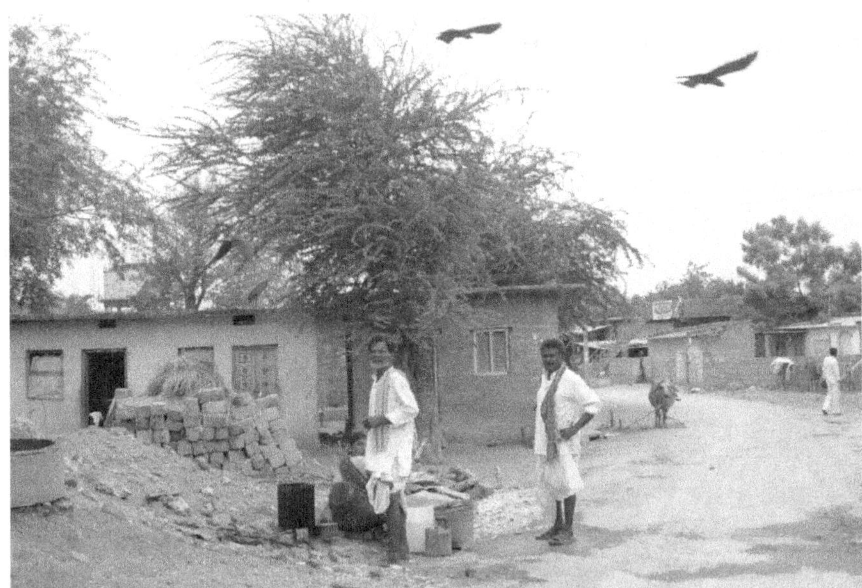

Indian Village

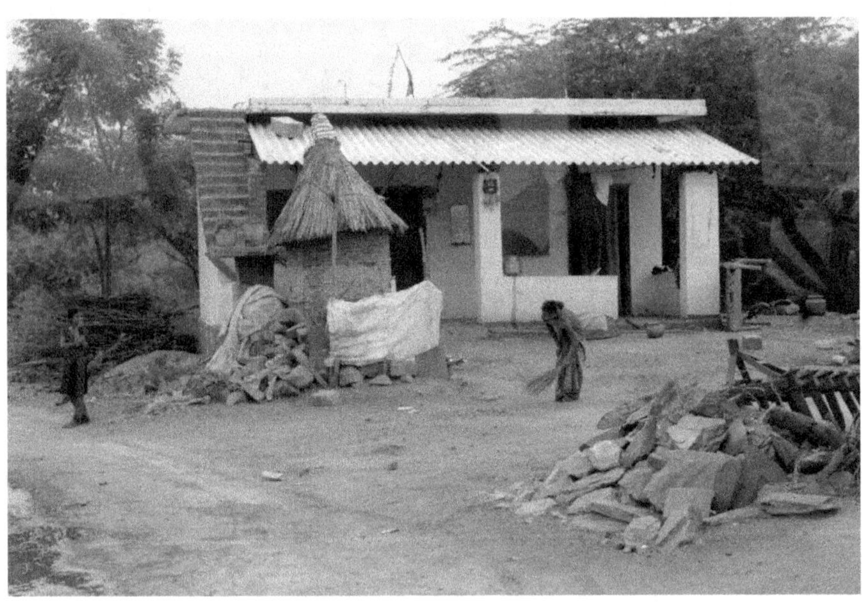

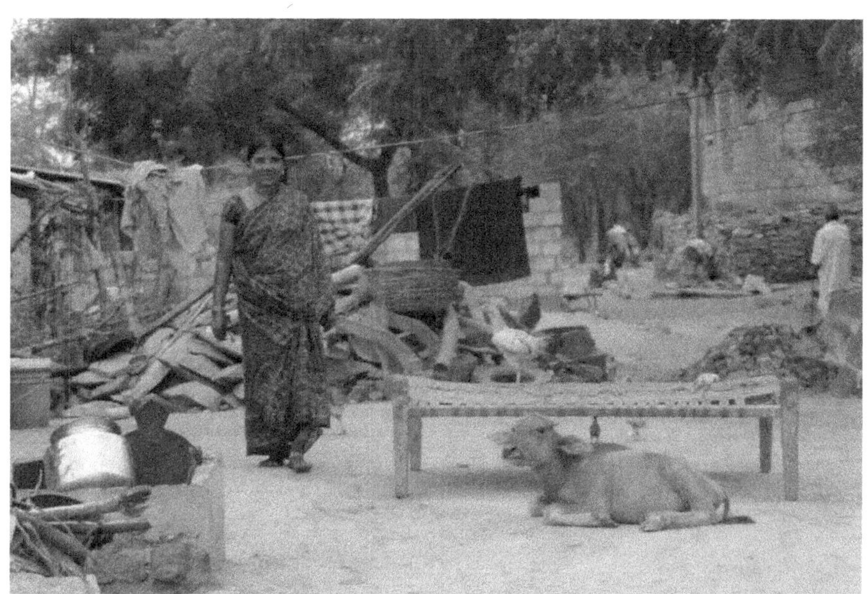

Indian Village

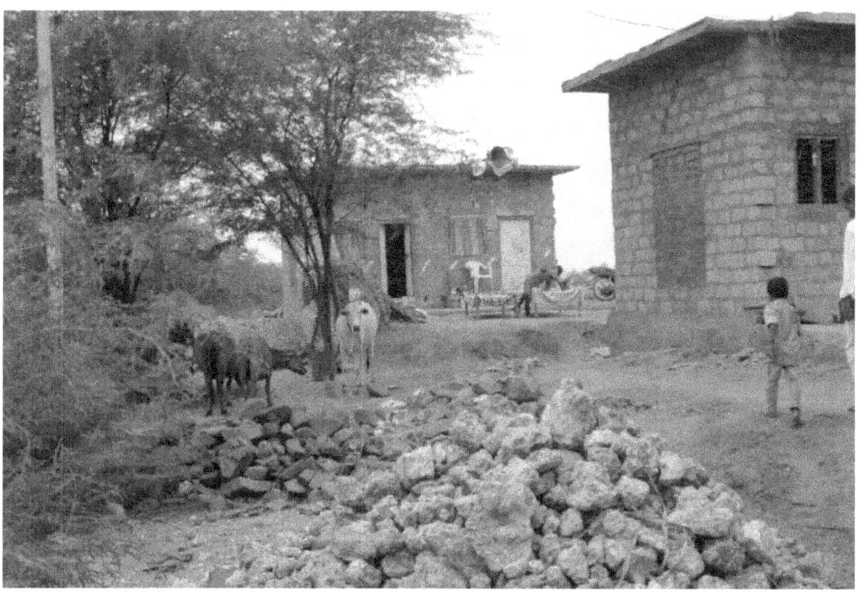

Indian Village

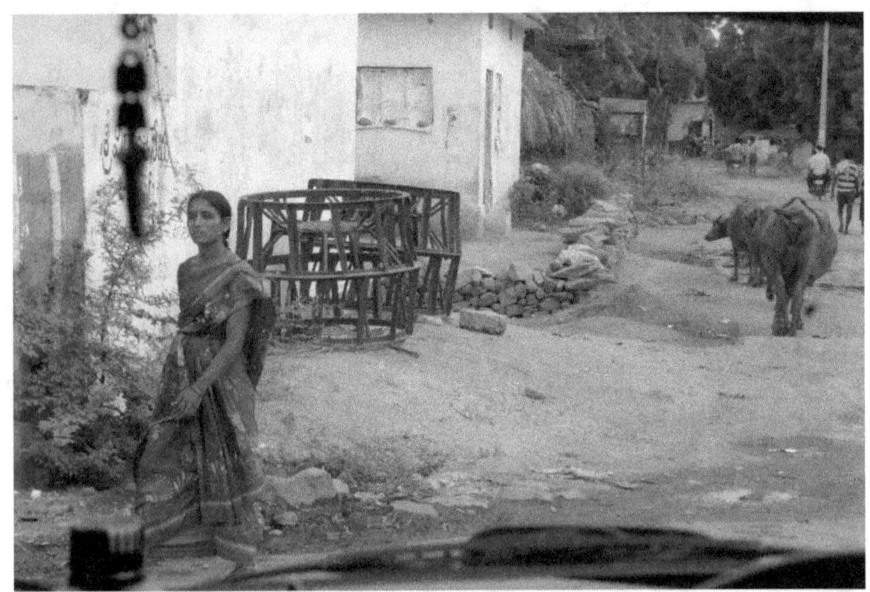

Indian Village

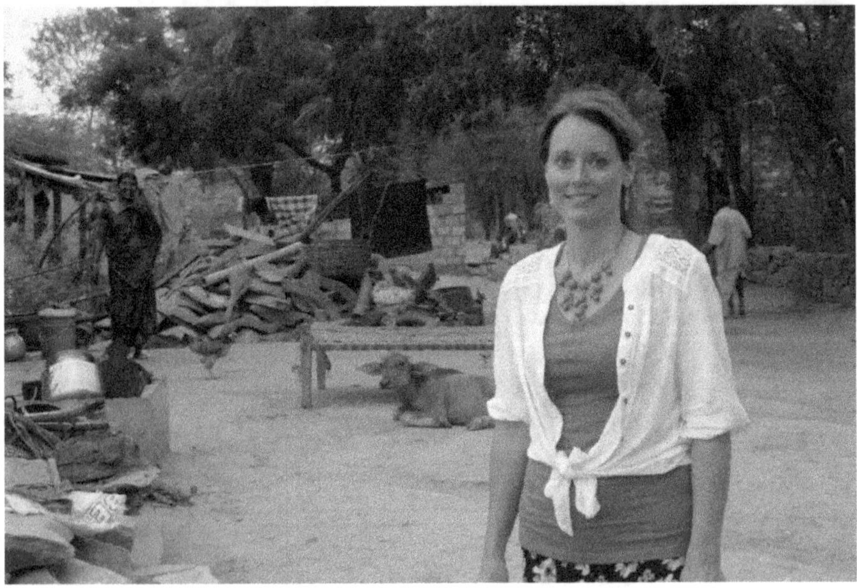

Indian Village

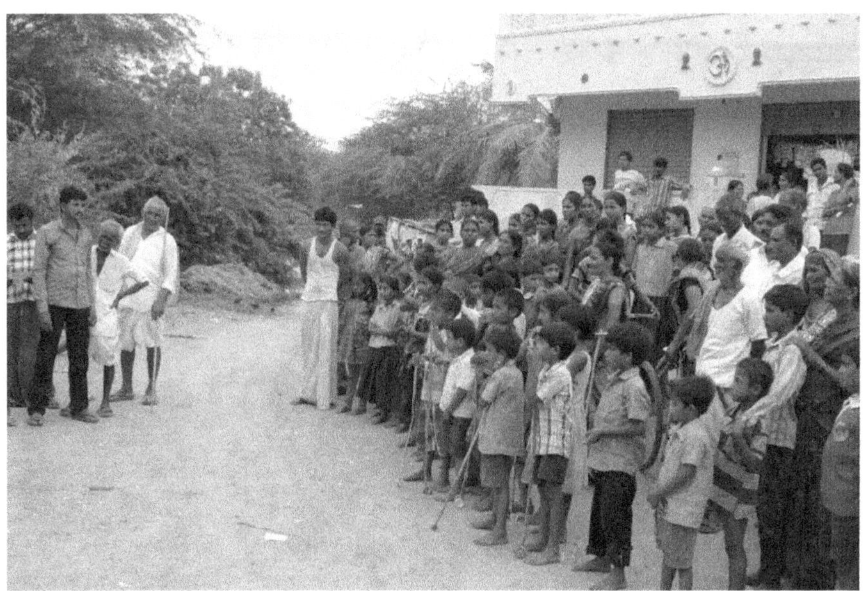

Indian Village

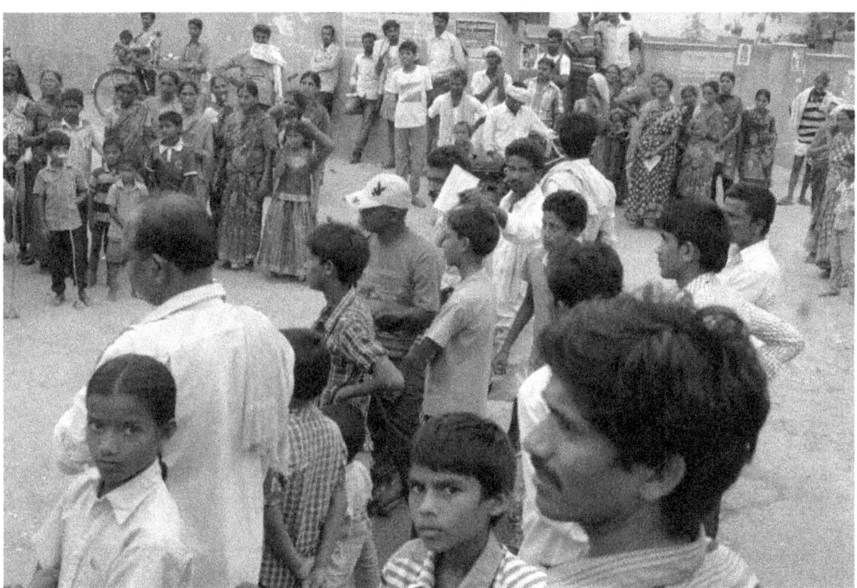

Indian Village

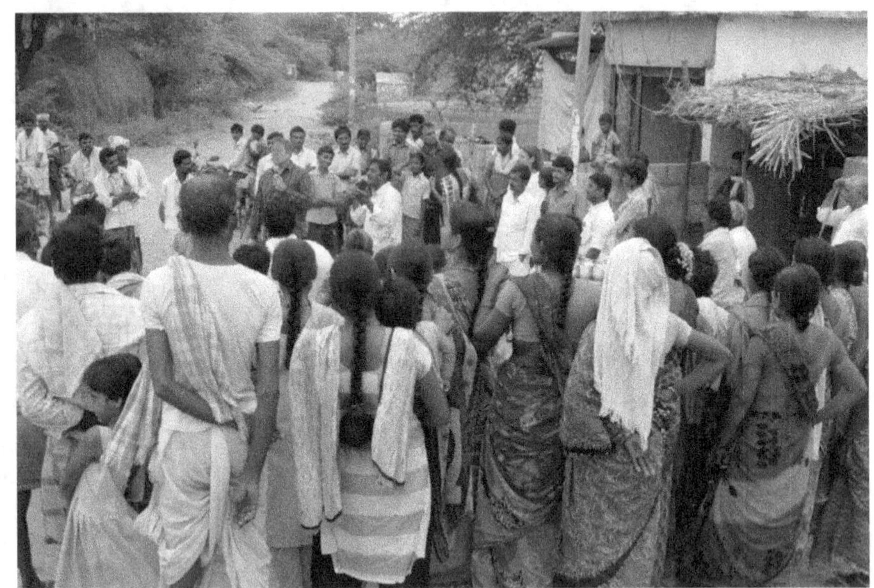

Joel preaching in an Indian Village

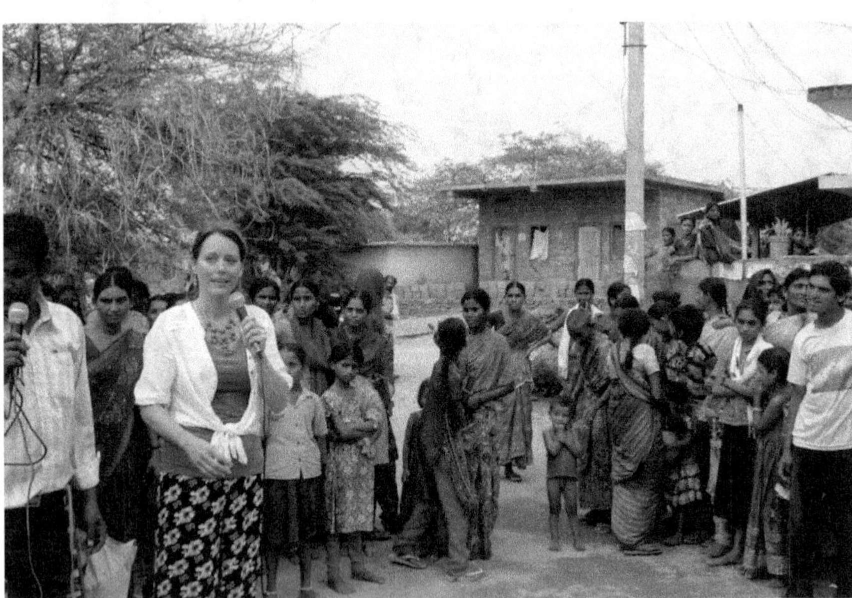

Heidi preaching in an Indian Village

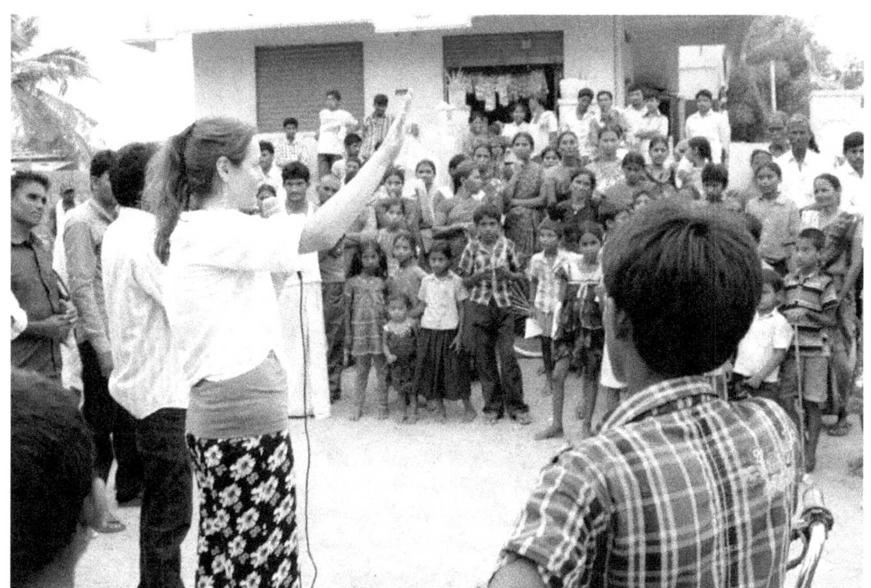

Heidi preaching in an Indian Village

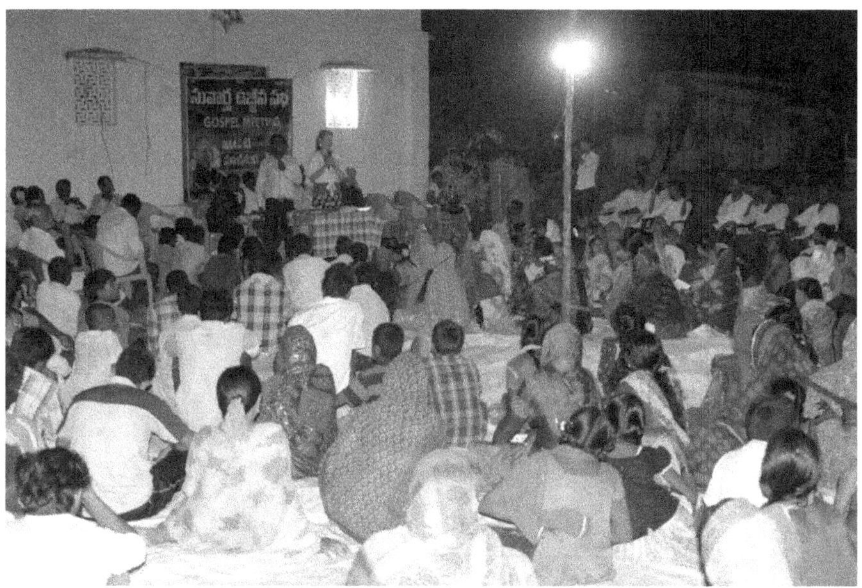

Heidi preaching in an Indian Village

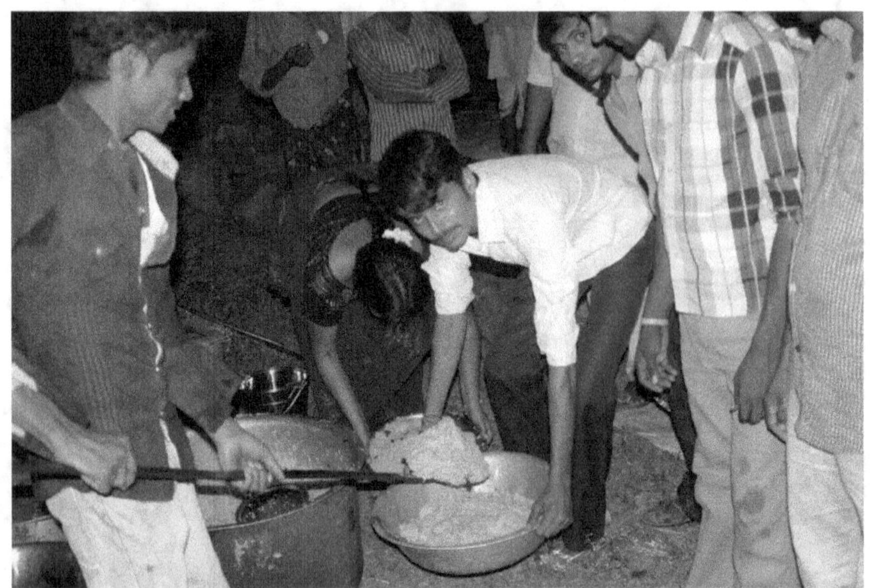

Indian Village

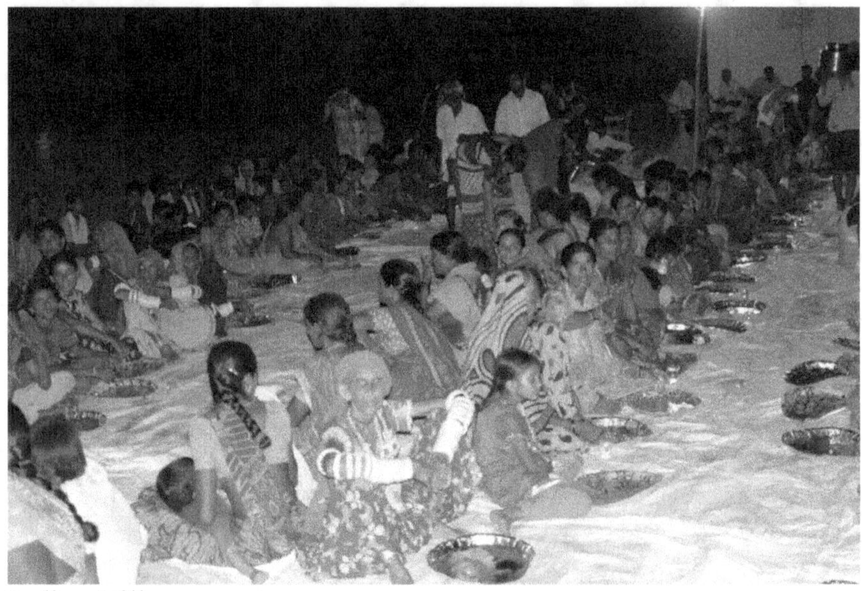

Indian Village

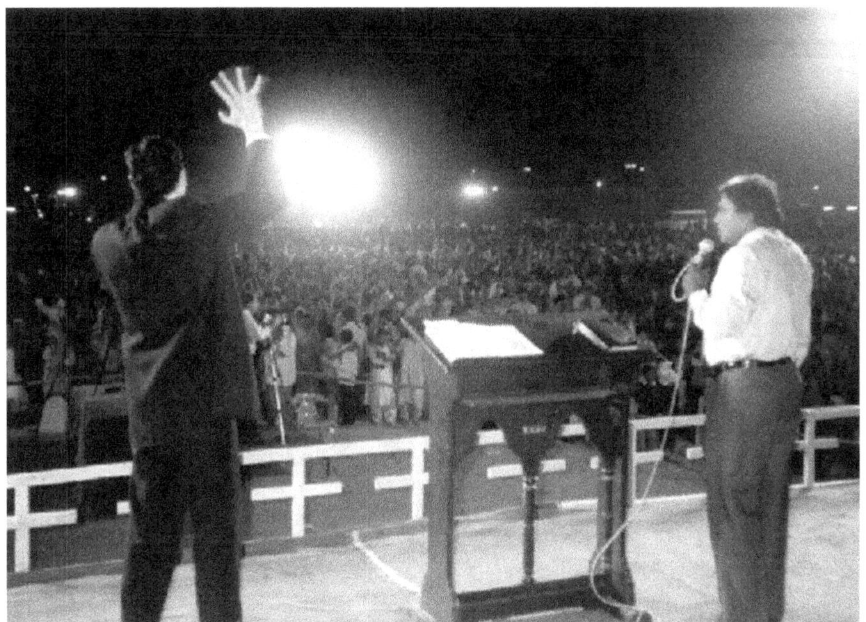

Warangal, India

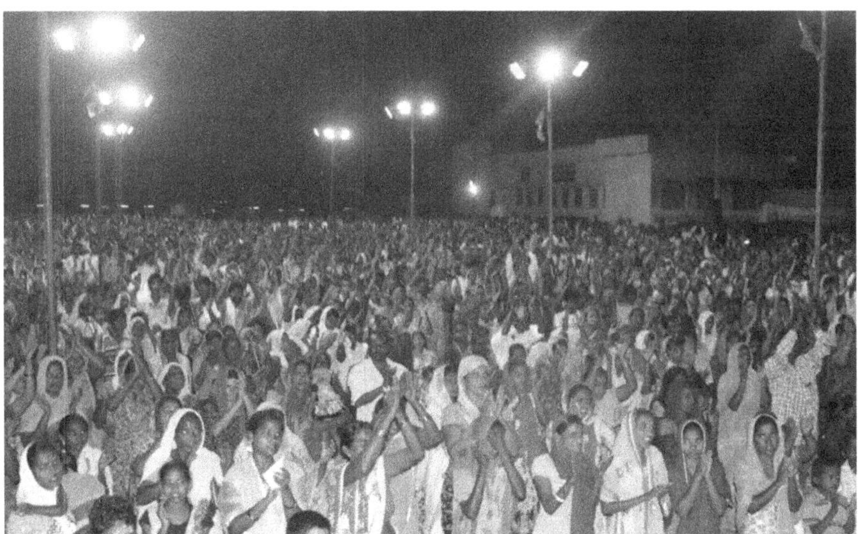

Suryapet, India

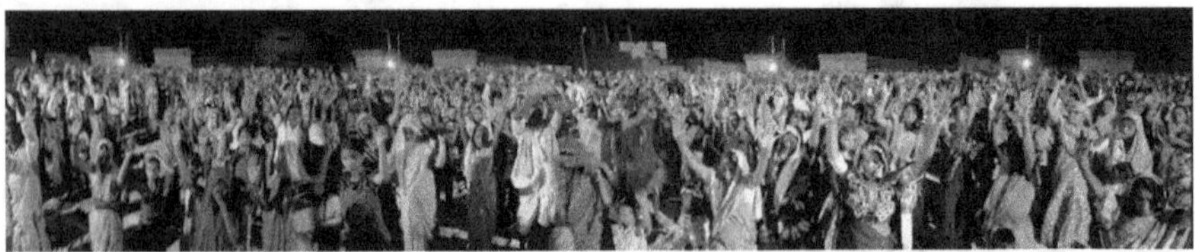

Huzurnagar, India

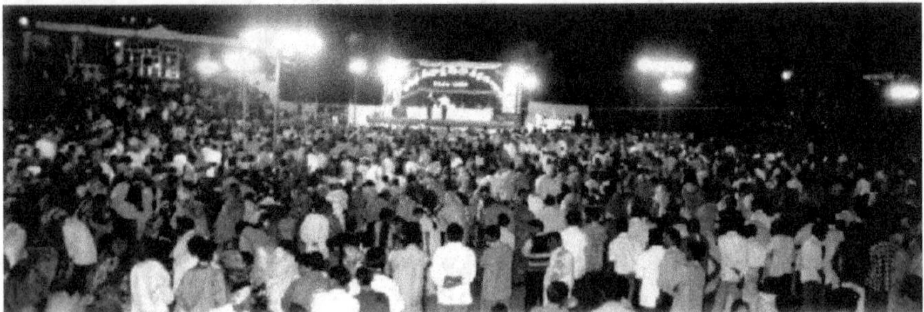

Warangal, India

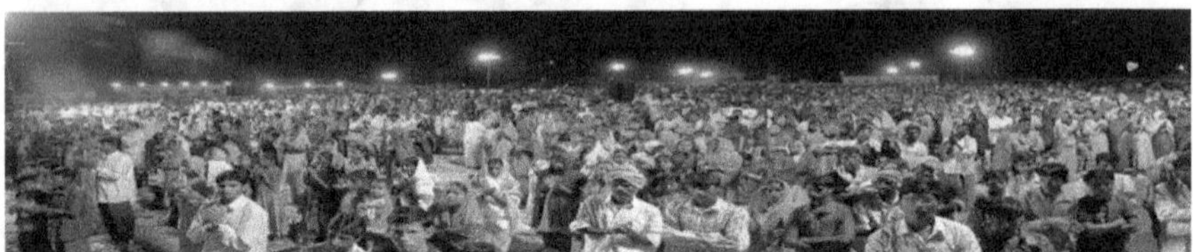

Miryalguda, India

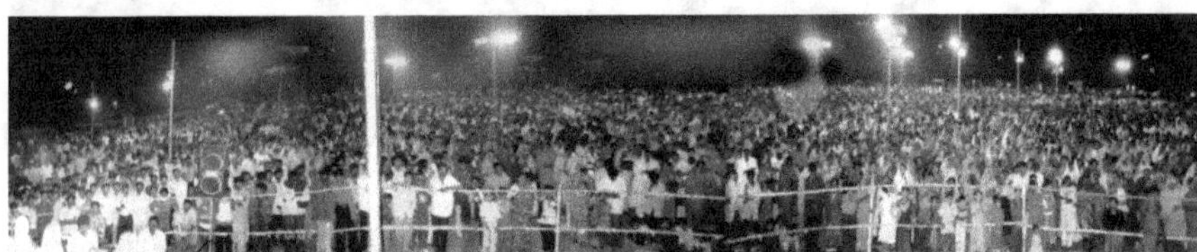

Kothagudem, India

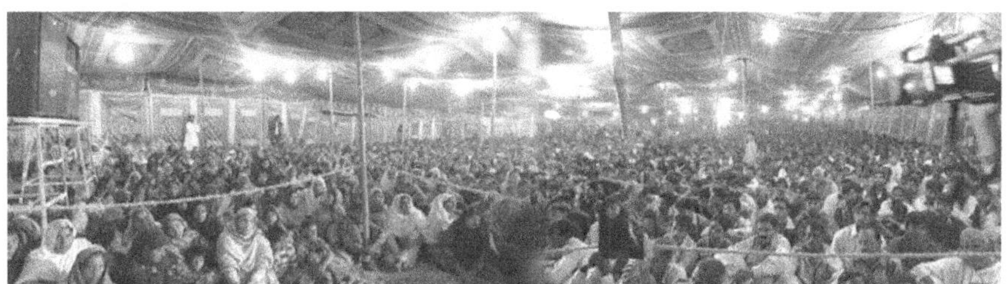

Sialkot, Pakistan

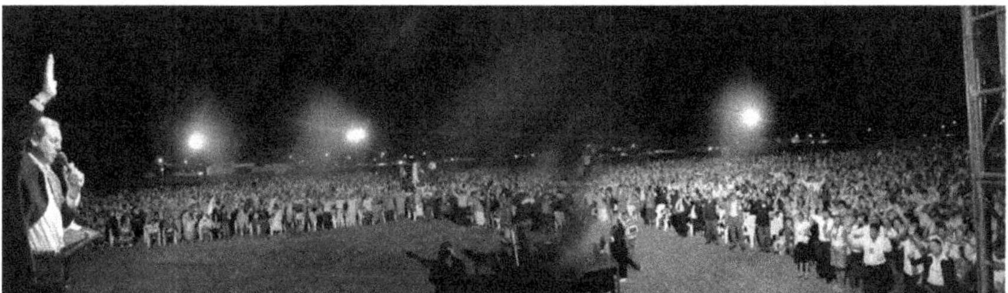

Tucupita, Venezuela

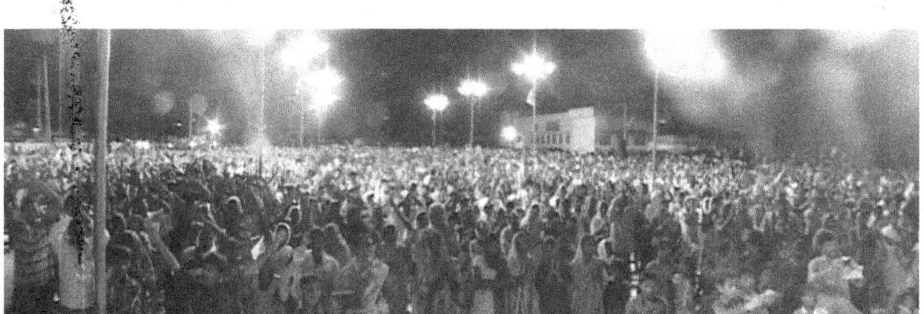

Suryapet, India

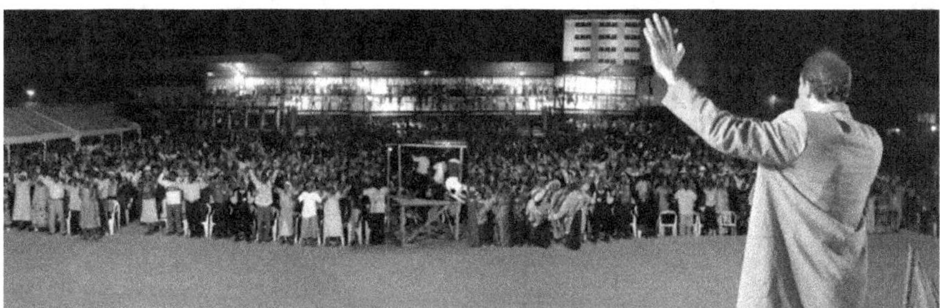

Douala, Cameroon

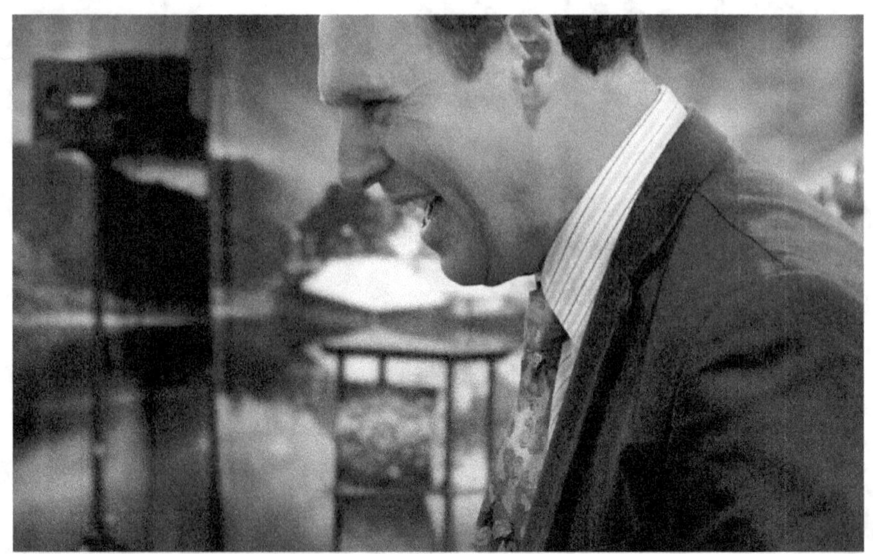

Joel Hitchcock, Delaware – USA

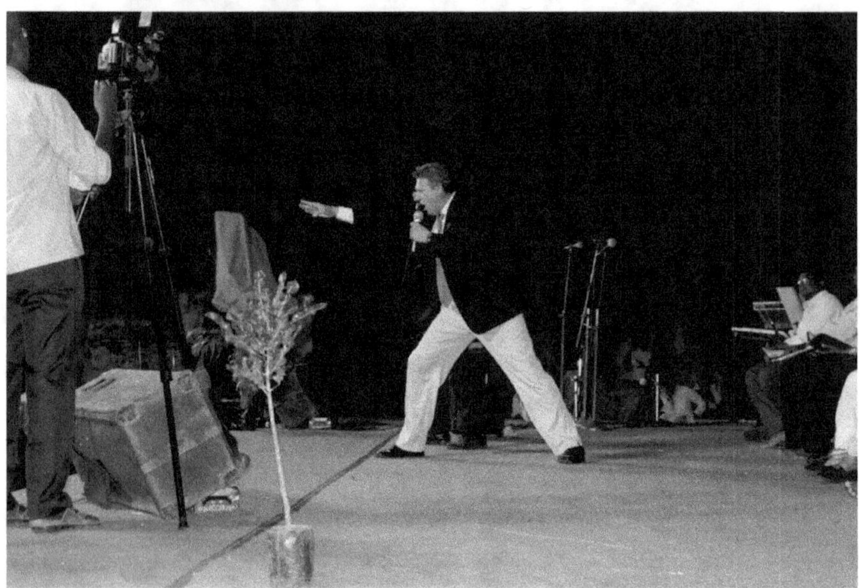

Joel Hitchcock – Suryapet, India

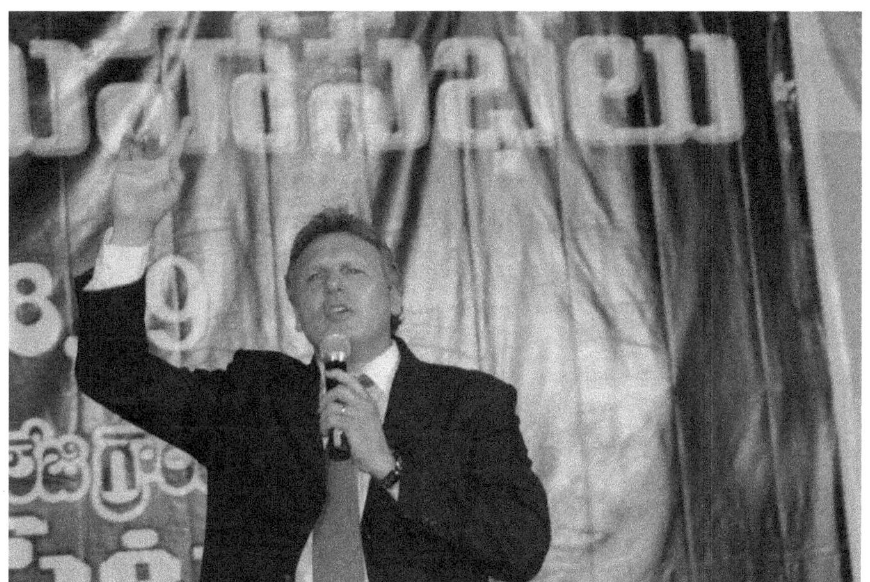

Joel Hitchcock – Suryapet, India

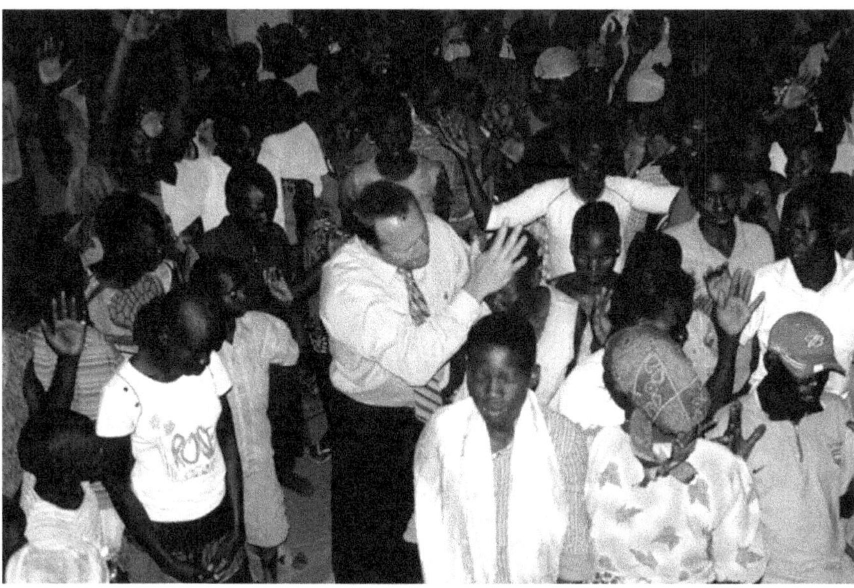

Joel Hitchcock – Gulu, Uganda

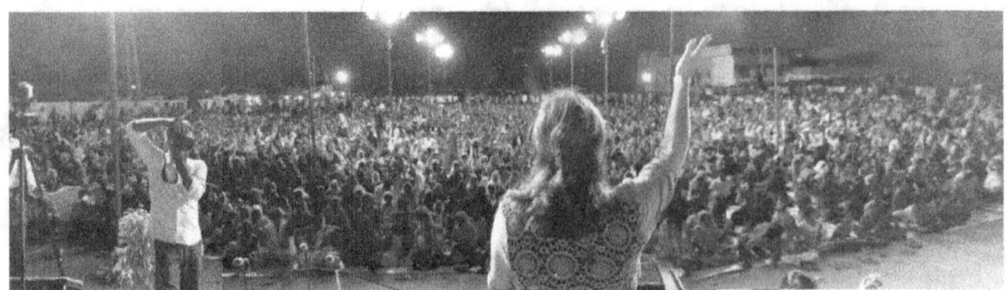

Heidi in India

Contact Information

Joel Hitchcock Ministries,

PO Box 936, Georgetown DE 19947

United States of America

302-858-0887

www.joelhitchcock.blogspot.com

www.youtube.com/joelhitchcock

www.twitter.com/joelhitchcock

www.facebook.com/hitchcockjoel

Dr. Joel Hitchcock has been in the full-time ministry for over 30 years as an evangelist and pastor.

Joel is married to Heidi and they have four children - Anthony, Rebekah, Timothy and Trey.

Joel has preached the Good News of Salvation, Healing and the Holy Spirit all around the world - in more than 45 countries. Multitudes have attended his mass evangelism miracle campaigns.

Joel has authored several full-sized books such as:

- Son of God and Man – the Deity and Humanity of Jesus Christ;
- Christ in you – Experience the Power of Oneness with God;

- The Miracle Ministry of Signs and Wonders;
- Mass Evangelism – the Power of City-Wide Gospel Campaigns;
- Miracles for the Multitudes (Combination of the Miracle and Mass Evangelism books)
- Praying and Proclaiming God's Abundant Provision;
- Praying and Proclaiming God's Abundant Provision (for women);
- Young Fire - End Time Youth Revivalists for the Great Awakening;
- Divine Romance - God and His Beloved in the Song of Songs;
- Your Daughters Shall Prophesy - an affirmation of Women's Ministry (Teaching, Preaching, and Leadership);

Joel has also authored several smaller booklets such as:

- The Great King and the Little Ant;
- One Almighty Mediator; and
- When Jesus Moves into your House
- The Divine Healing Prayer

Joel also maintains several blogs, and has a growing YouTube ministry, such as:

- www.joelhitchcock.blogspot.com
- www.youtube.com/joelhitchcock

Having completed is doctoral thesis on *The Deity and Humanity of Jesus Christ,* Joel's great passion is centered around the Person of Jesus Christ, and our union with Him.

Heidi Hitchcock was born and raised in Delaware. After High School, she attended Bob Jones and Liberty University, where she graduated.

She also furthered her Biblical studies at the *World College of Theology.*

Together with her husband Joel she has traveled and spread the Gospel to many states in the USA, several countries in Africa, Venezuela in South America, and India. With Joel, she co-pastors *River City Church* in Rehoboth DE. Heidi loves the Lord and people, and has a passion to lead people into a real relationship with God.